Gardening with Grandma

An Alzheimer's Story for Children and Their Families

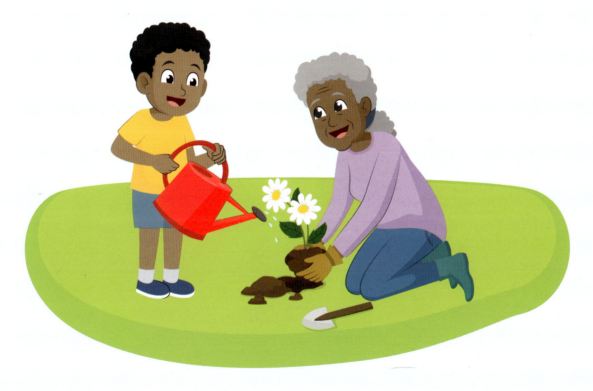

Story by
Linda Bozzo

Illustrated by
Mudassir M. Abid

Published by

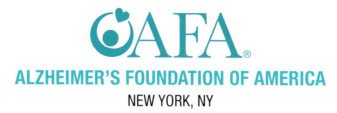

ALZHEIMER'S FOUNDATION OF AMERICA
NEW YORK, NY

ISBN: 978-1-7354076-2-3

Story by Linda Bozzo
Illustrations by Mudassir M. Abid

Layout by Gary A. Rosenberg
www.garyarosenberg.com

Printed in the United States of America

Each spring, Luke looked forward to gardening with Grandma in her yard next door.

He loved learning about different types of flowers and plants and watching them grow during their special time together.

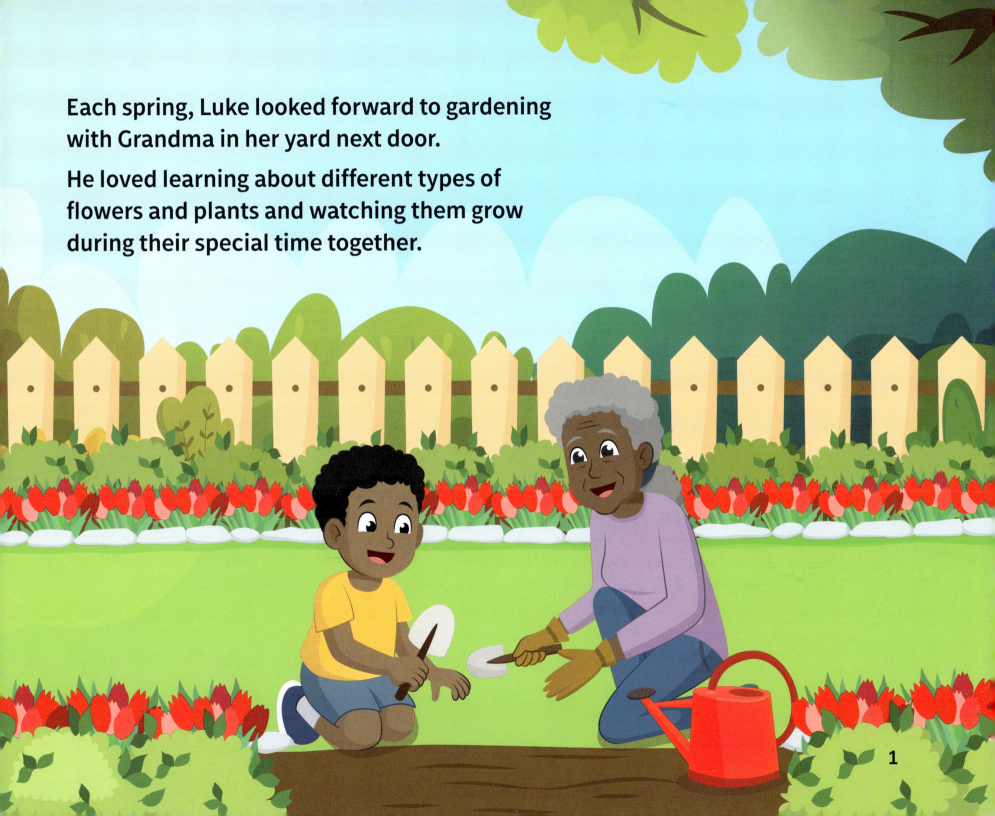

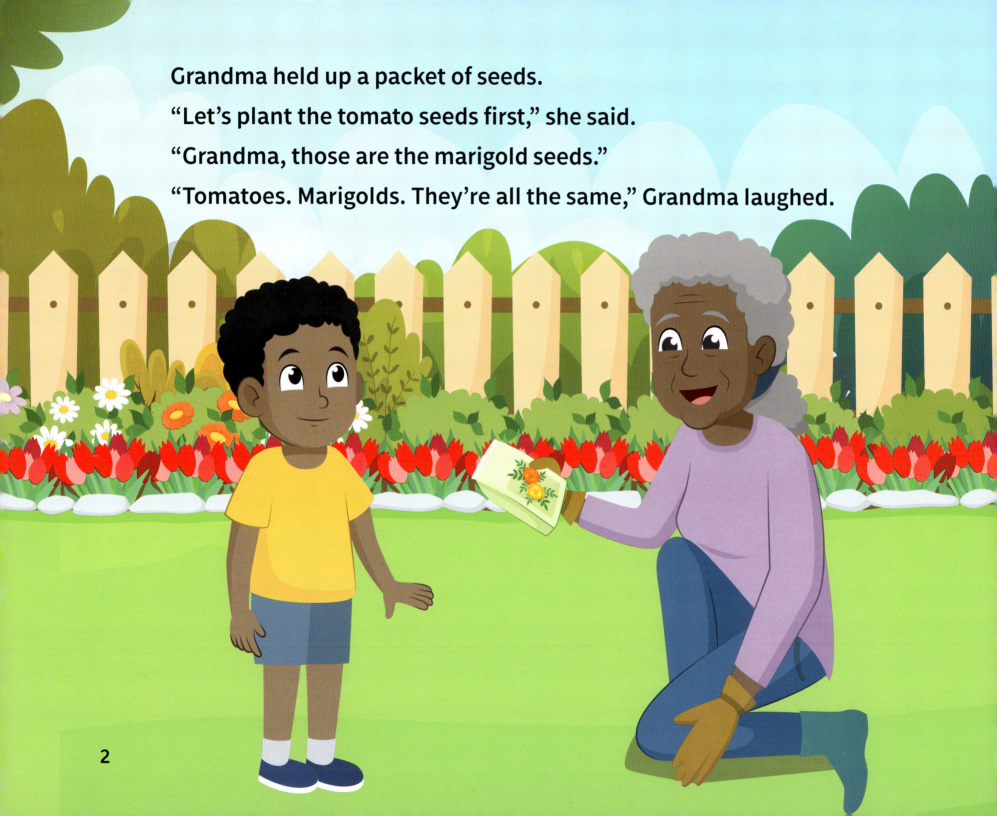

Grandma held up a packet of seeds.

"Let's plant the tomato seeds first," she said.

"Grandma, those are the marigold seeds."

"Tomatoes. Marigolds. They're all the same," Grandma laughed.

2

Luke dug shallow holes.
Grandma dropped in the seeds.

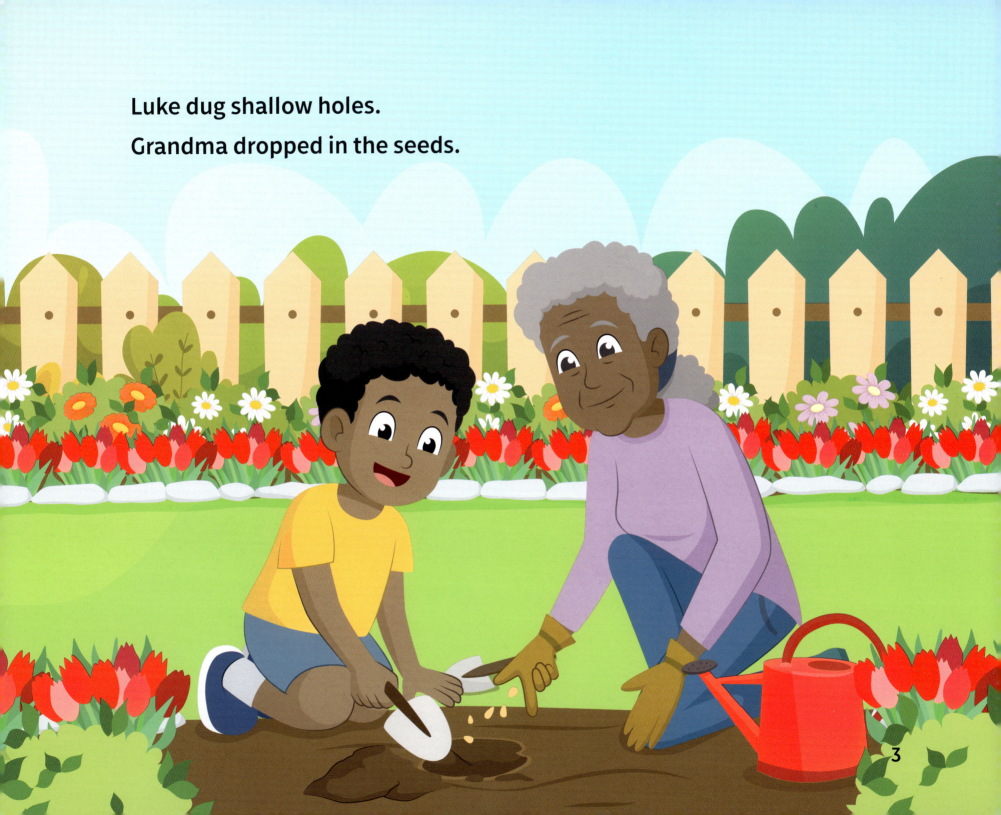

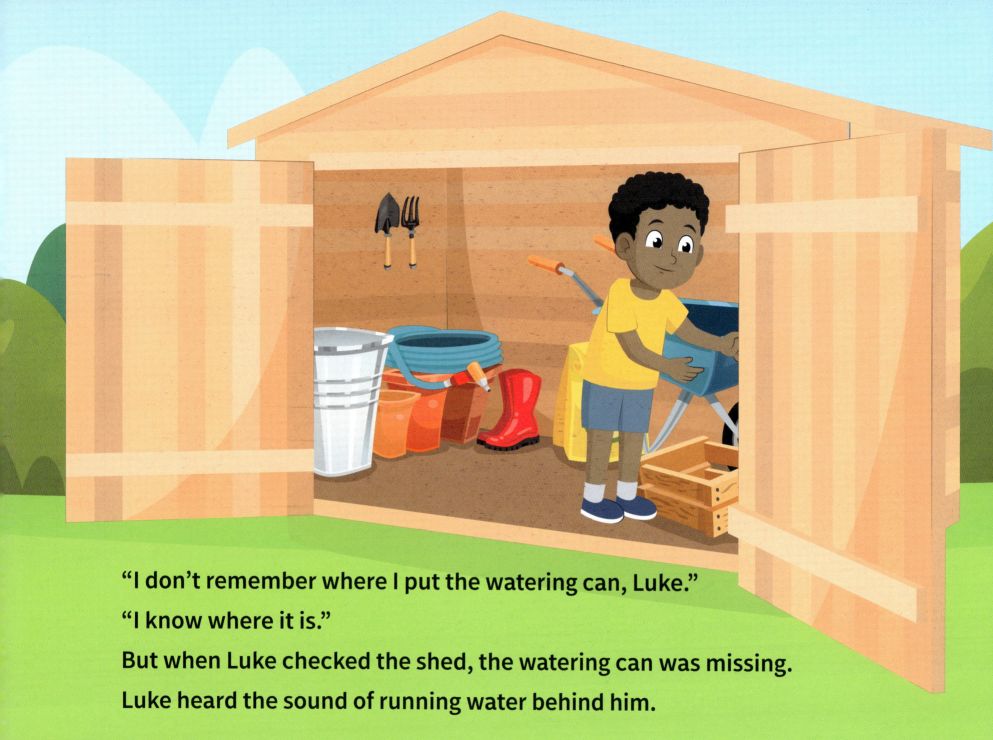

"I don't remember where I put the watering can, Luke."

"I know where it is."

But when Luke checked the shed, the watering can was missing.

Luke heard the sound of running water behind him.

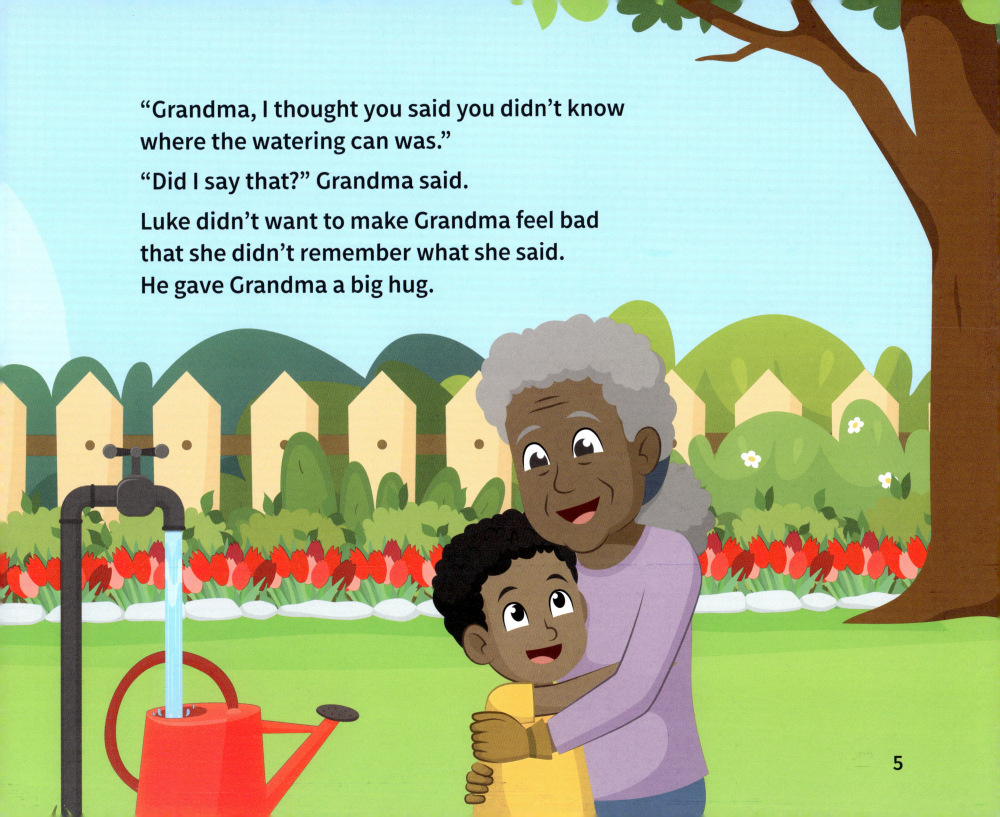

"Grandma, I thought you said you didn't know where the watering can was."

"Did I say that?" Grandma said.

Luke didn't want to make Grandma feel bad that she didn't remember what she said. He gave Grandma a big hug.

That night, Luke told his parents he was starting to feel worried about Grandma.

When Luke mentioned the watering can, Mom told him, "Try to be patient with Grandma when she forgets or gets confused. She's been having some trouble remembering things."

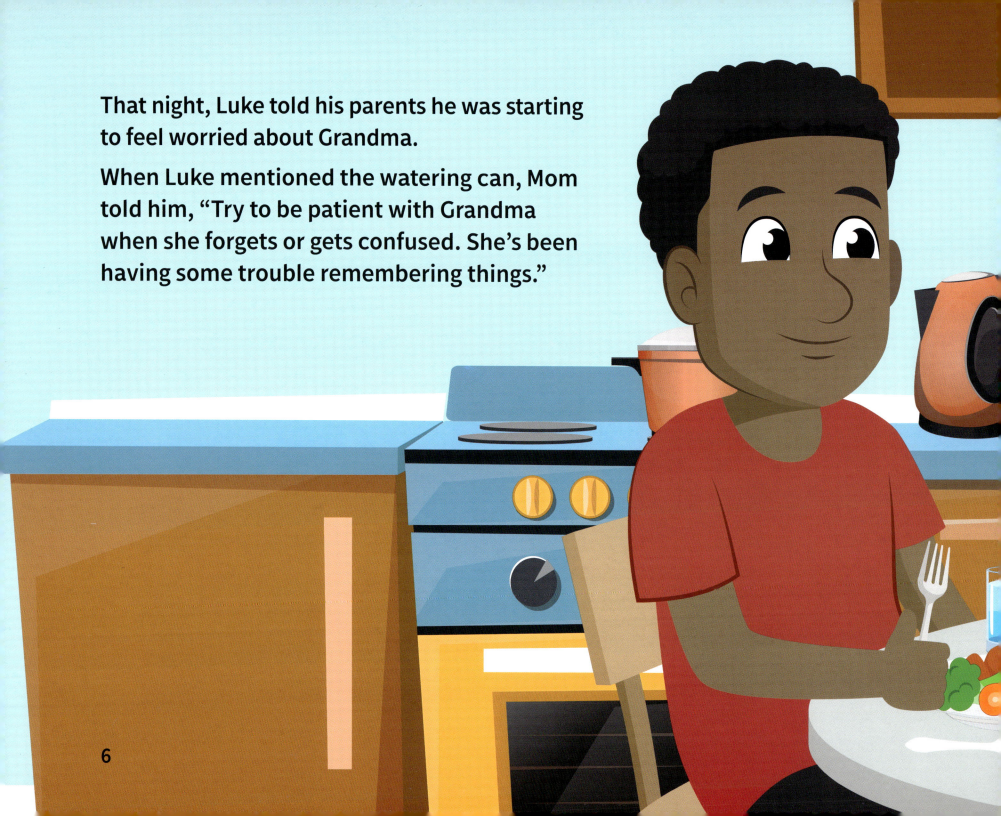

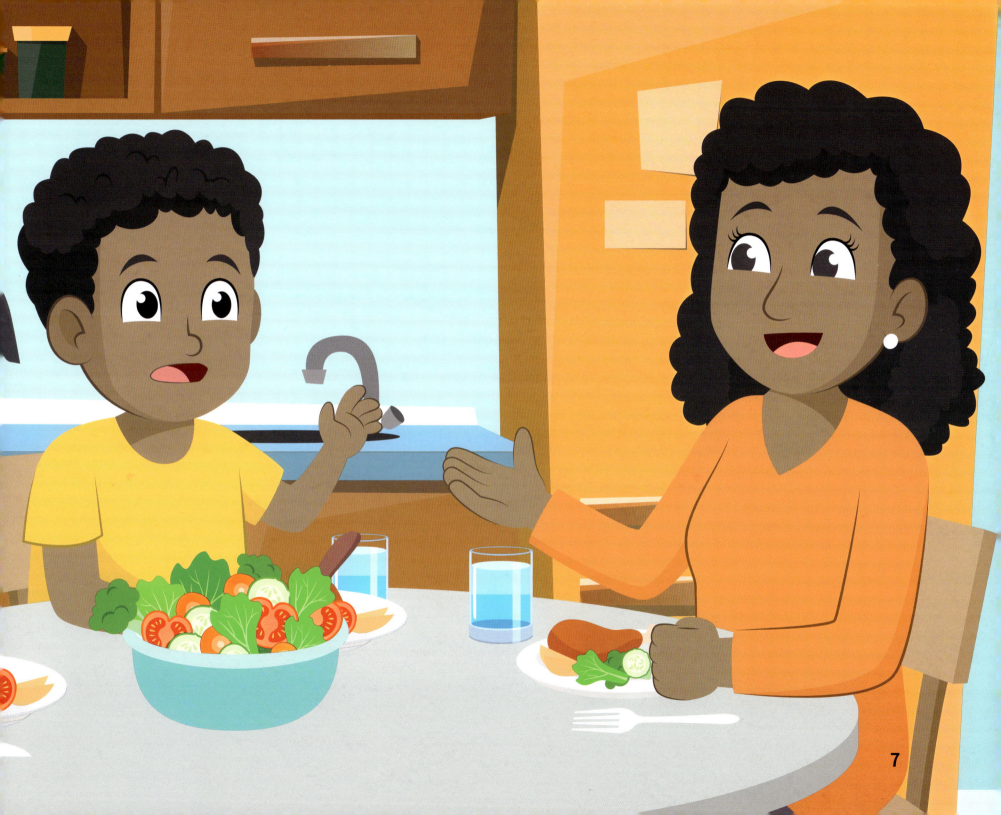

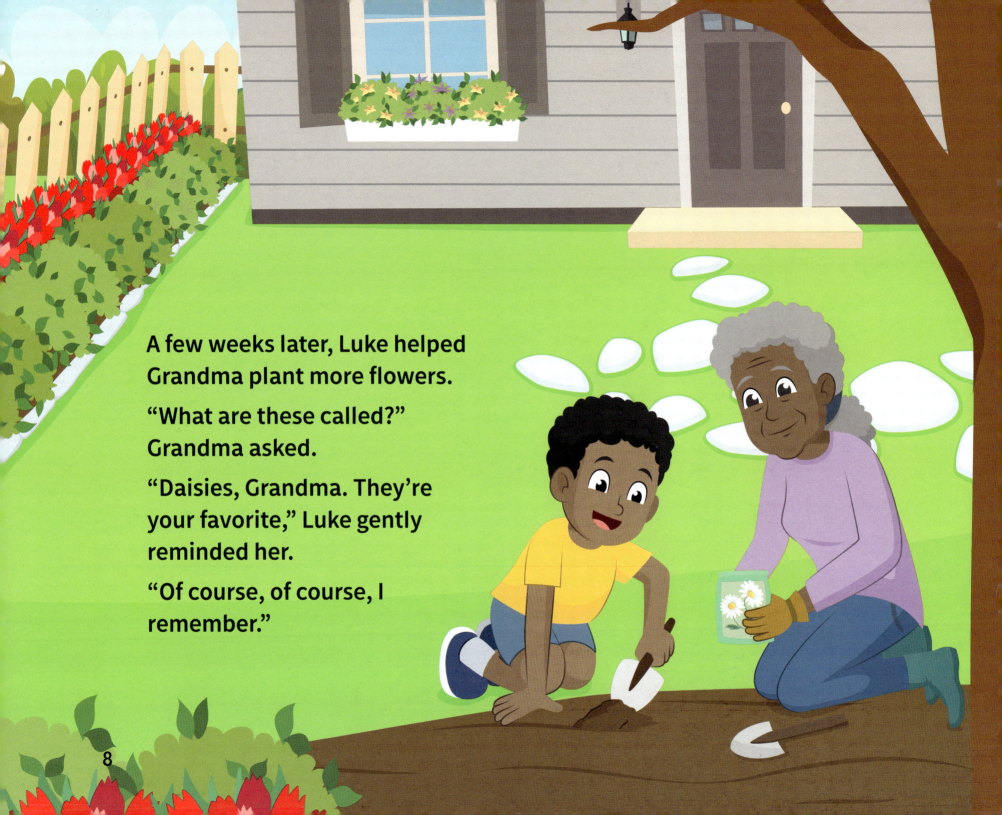

A few weeks later, Luke helped Grandma plant more flowers.

"What are these called?" Grandma asked.

"Daisies, Grandma. They're your favorite," Luke gently reminded her.

"Of course, of course, I remember."

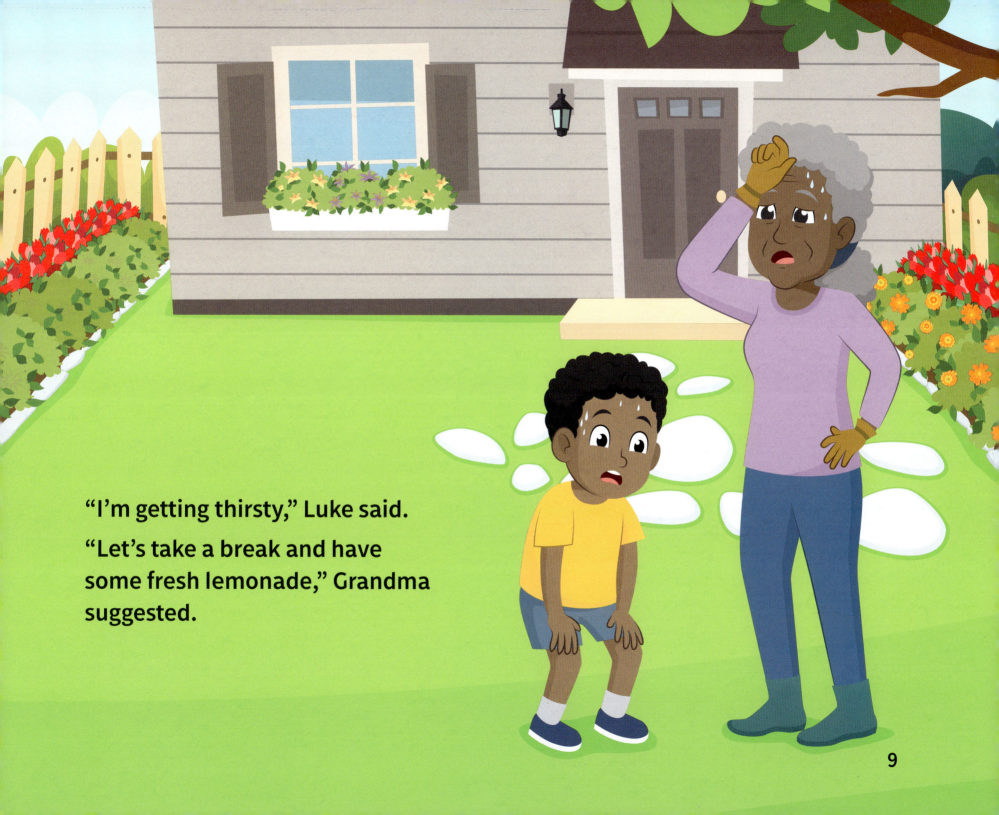

"I'm getting thirsty," Luke said.

"Let's take a break and have some fresh lemonade," Grandma suggested.

9

Inside, Luke found dirty dishes piled high in the sink.

Grandma's kitchen was usually tidy and clean.

"Grandma, what happened?"

"I didn't do that."

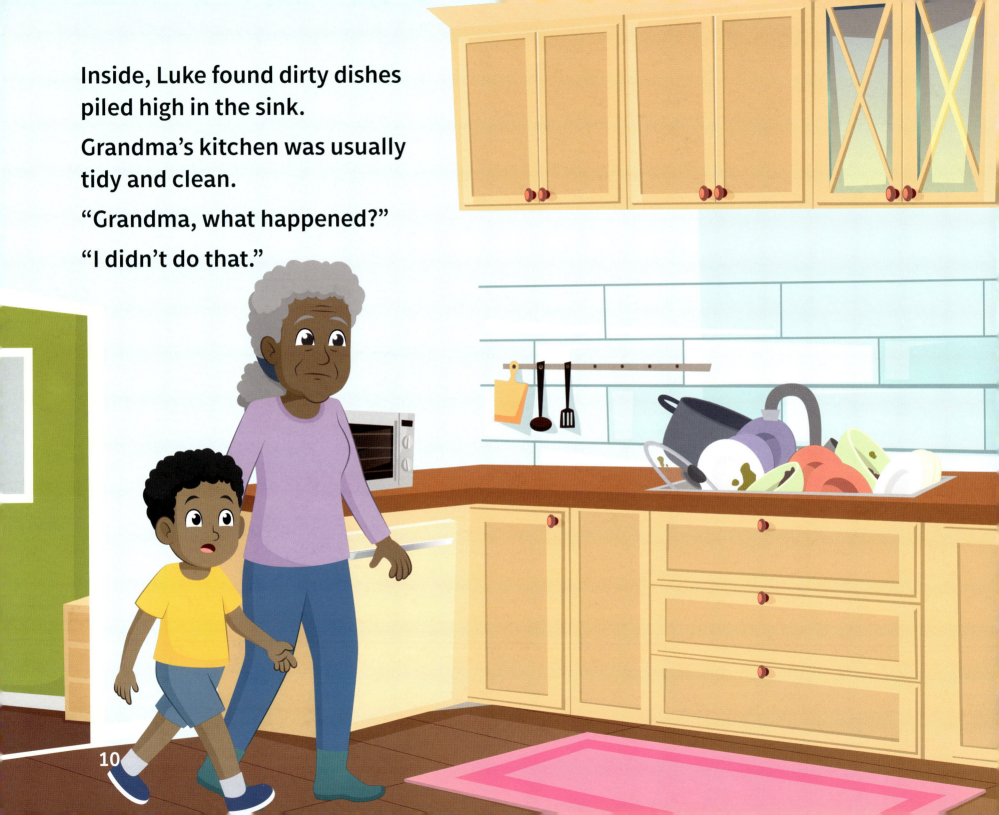

Luke knew it wasn't good to argue with Grandma. It would only upset her. He remembered it was best to do something that would make her happy instead.

So, Luke turned on some music.

Together they sang as Grandma washed the dishes and Luke dried them. Then he went home.

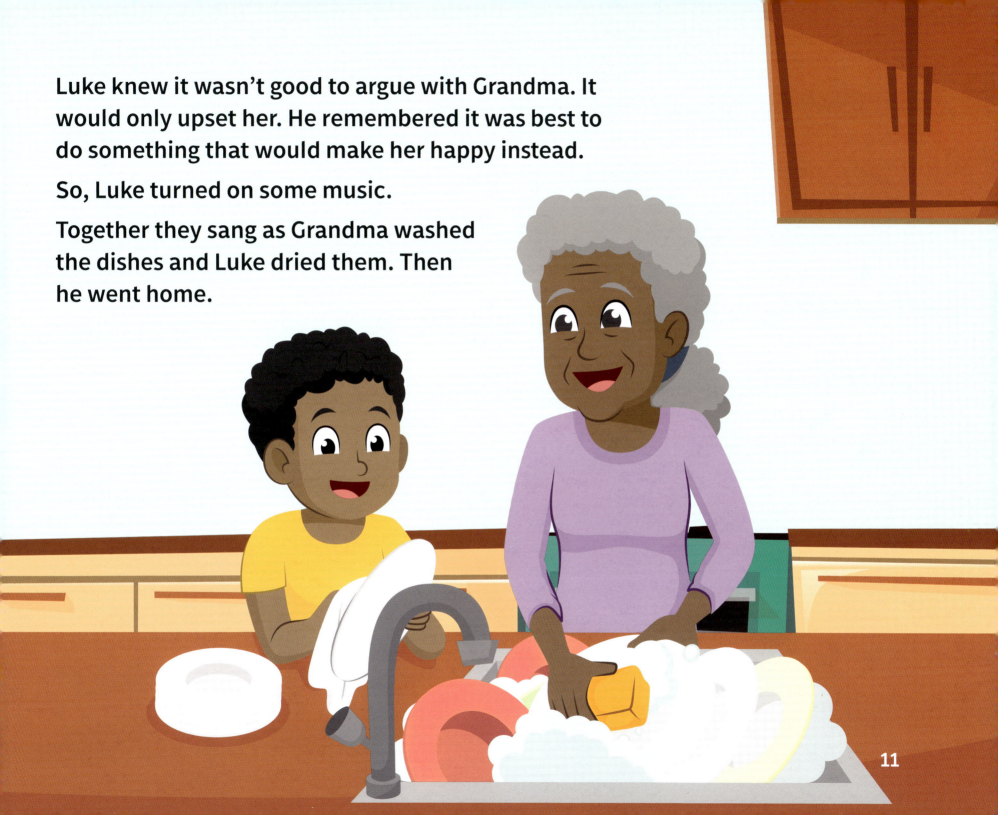

11

Over time, Grandma became confused more often and had trouble remembering things. Luke's mom took Grandma to the doctor for a check-up. Afterwards, they met as a family to explain some things to Luke.

"Grandma has Alzheimer's disease," said Mom.

"Over time, this can cause her to become confused and have trouble remembering."

"She doesn't look different," Luke said.

"Maybe not, but inside her brain is changing," Dad explained.

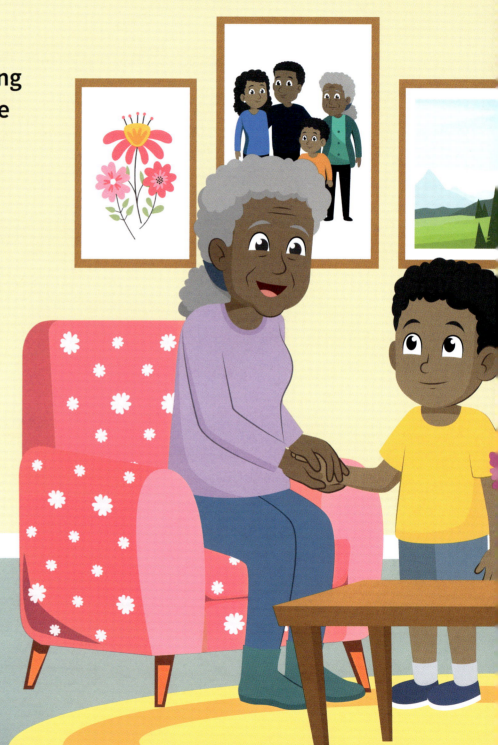

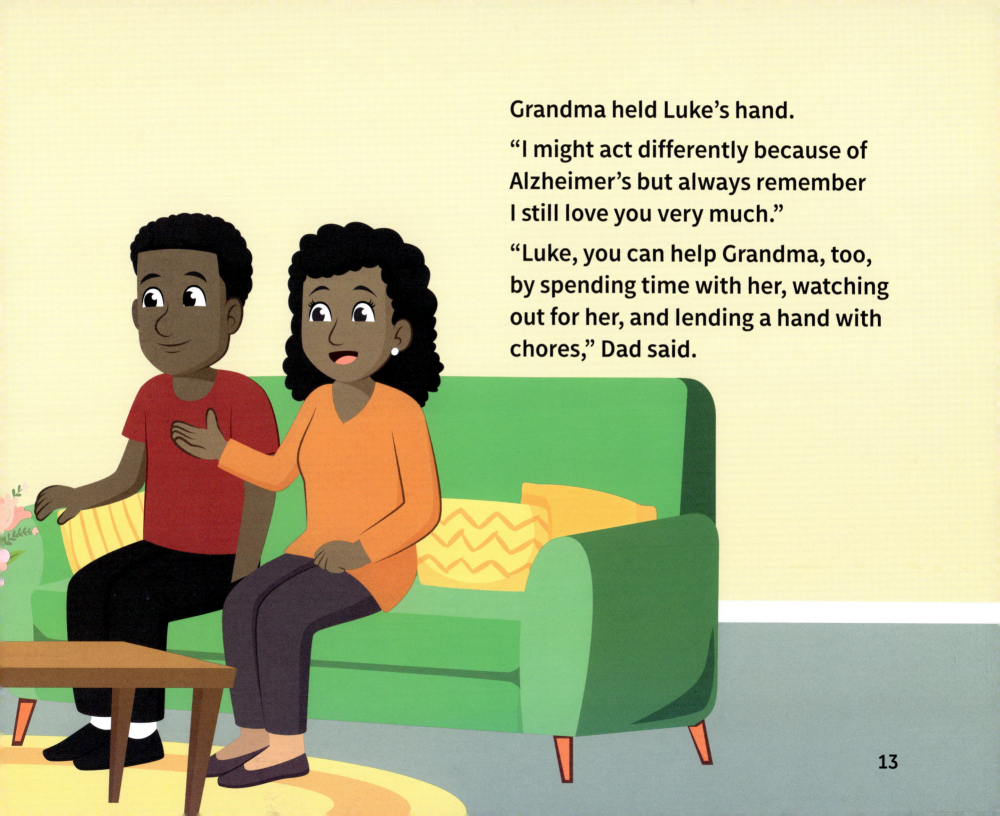

Grandma held Luke's hand.

"I might act differently because of Alzheimer's but always remember I still love you very much."

"Luke, you can help Grandma, too, by spending time with her, watching out for her, and lending a hand with chores," Dad said.

Luke and his parents helped Grandma every day, often bringing her groceries.

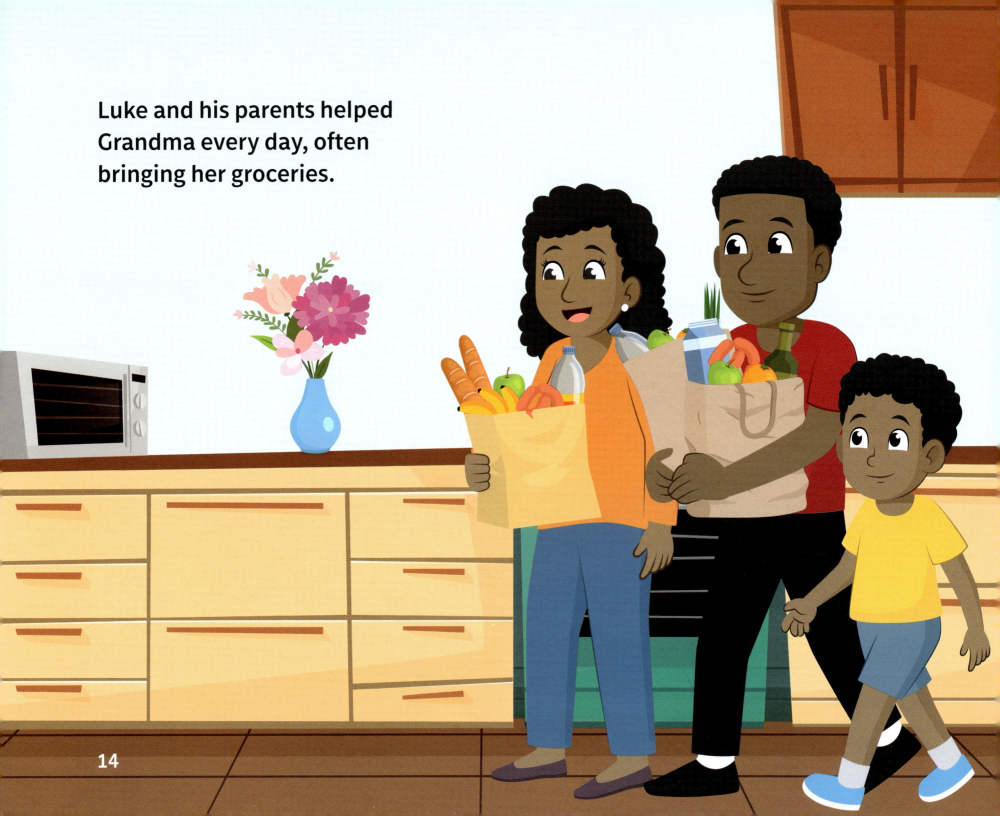

Then one summer day, Grandma told them proudly, "I weeded the garden!"

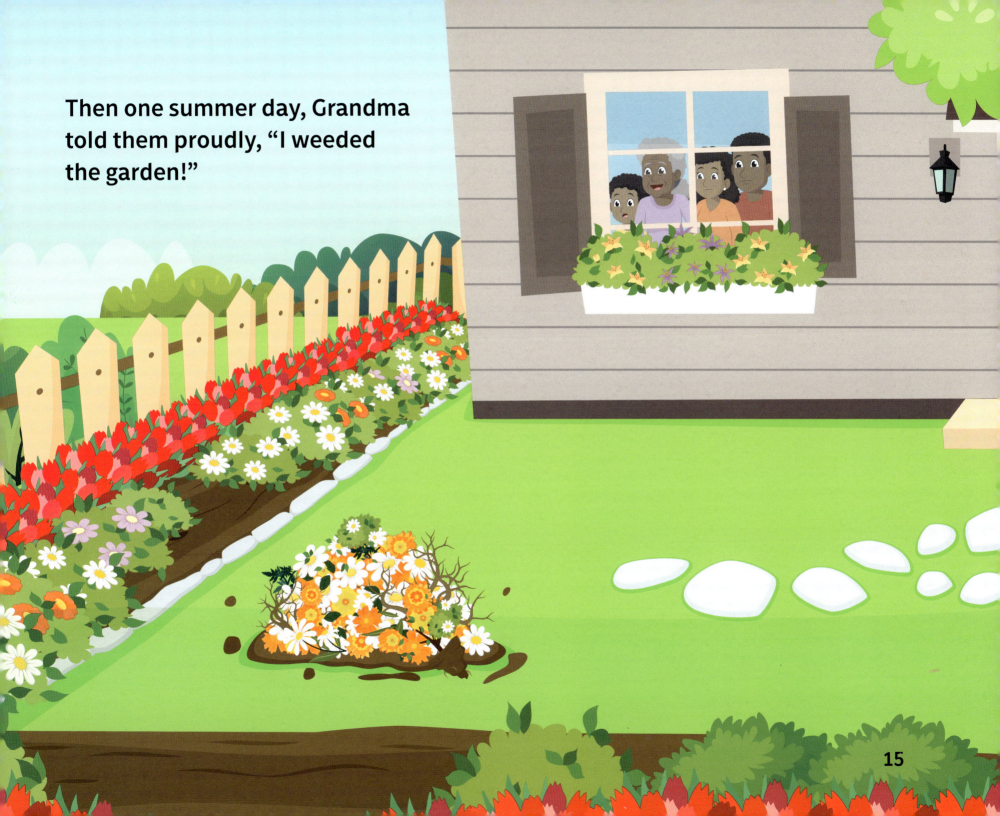

Dad helped Grandma inside while Luke and Mom replanted the flowers.

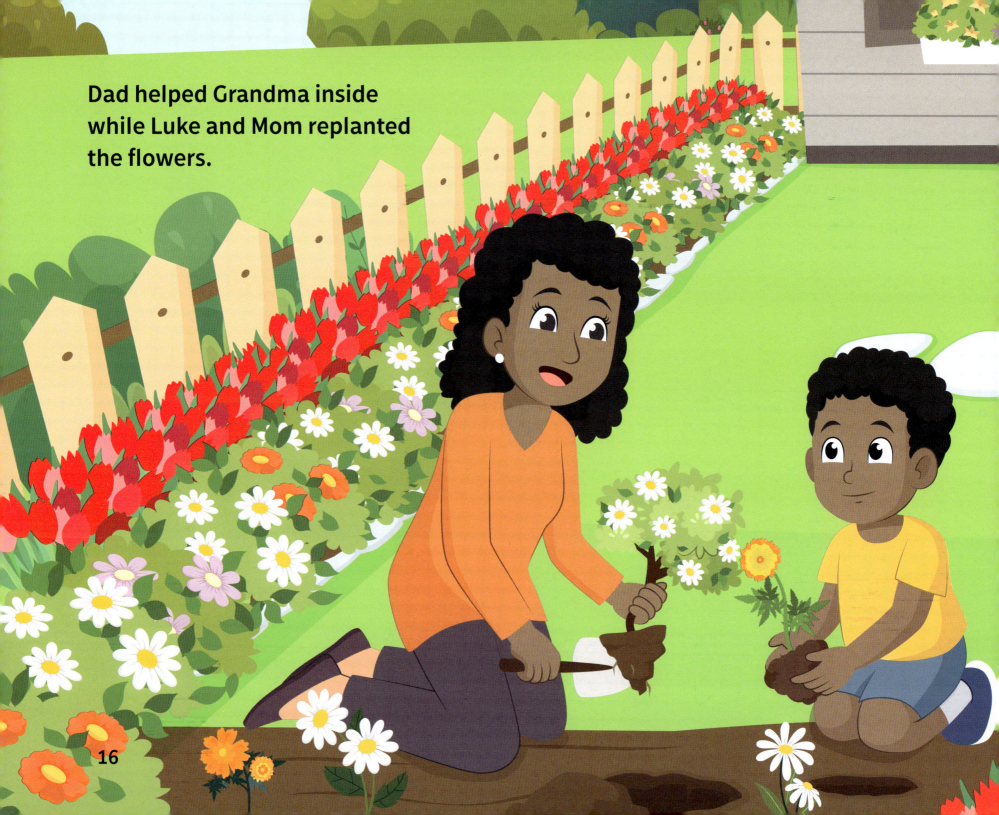

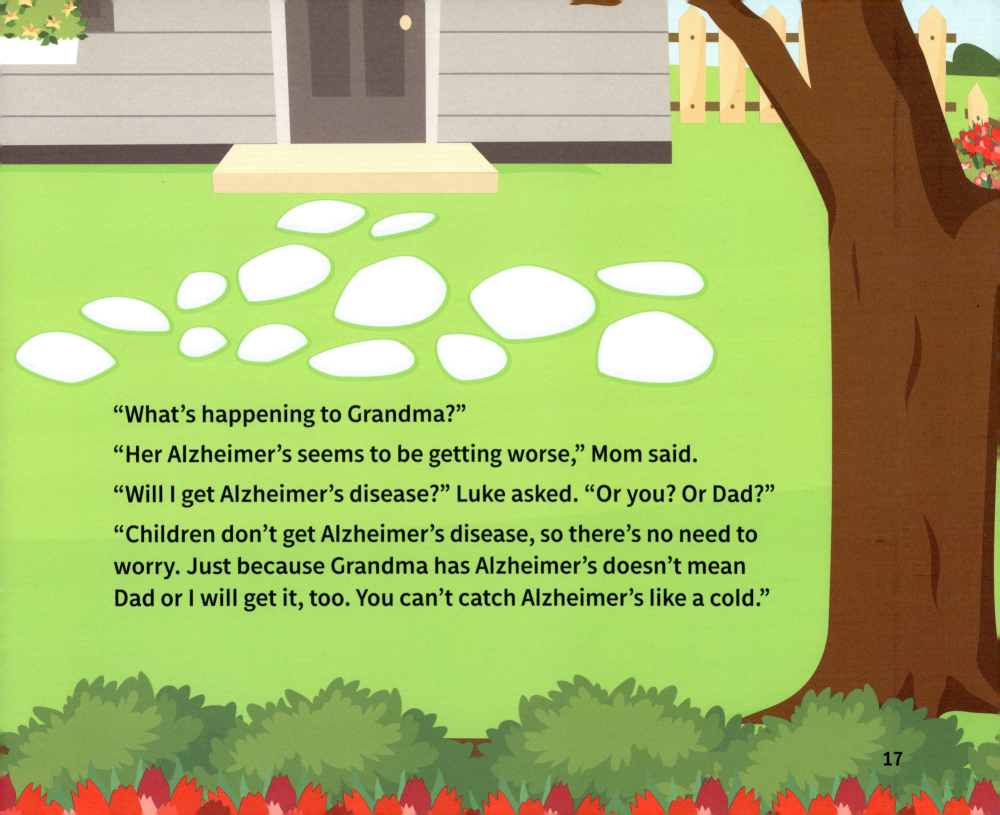

"What's happening to Grandma?"

"Her Alzheimer's seems to be getting worse," Mom said.

"Will I get Alzheimer's disease?" Luke asked. "Or you? Or Dad?"

"Children don't get Alzheimer's disease, so there's no need to worry. Just because Grandma has Alzheimer's doesn't mean Dad or I will get it, too. You can't catch Alzheimer's like a cold."

Then one day, mom explained, "The doctor thinks Grandma needs more help than we can give her. She thinks it would be best if we helped Grandma move to a new, smaller home that's easier for her. There will be adults called caregivers who are trained to help people with Alzheimer's, too."

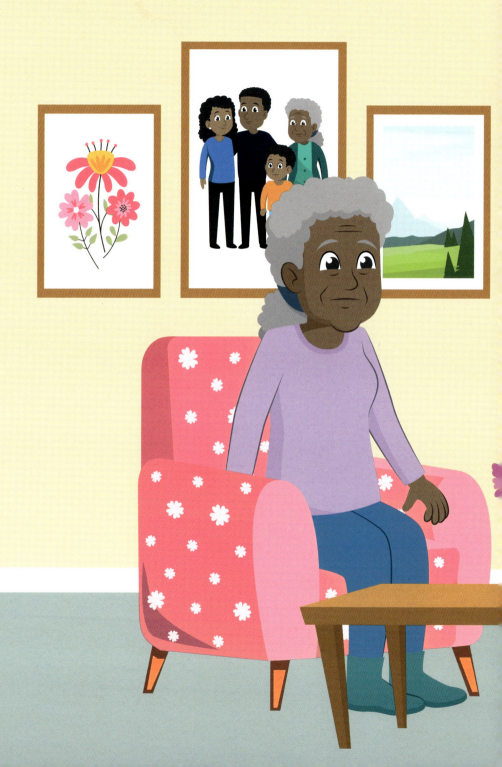

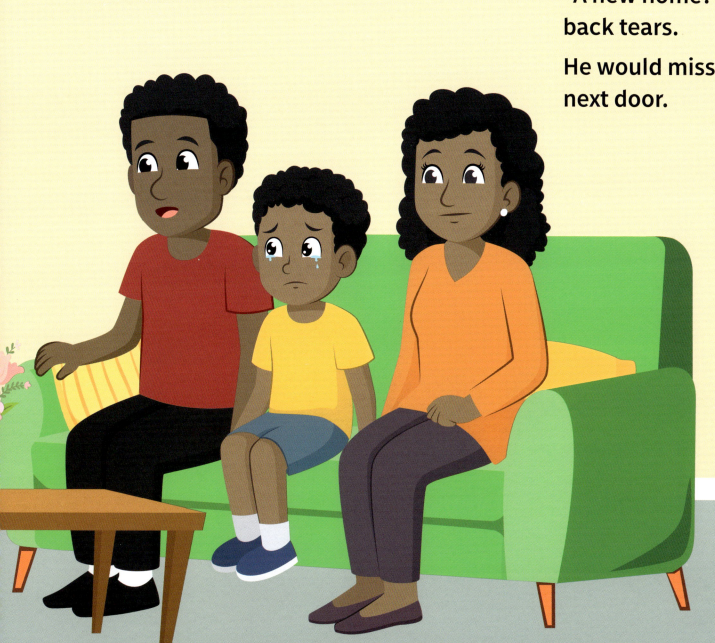

"A new home?" Luke choked back tears.

He would miss Grandma living next door.

"The doctor doesn't think I should live by myself anymore. My house is just too big for me to take care of. I'd really like to live somewhere that's cozy and comfortable," Grandma explained to Luke.

"The caregivers there will help keep Grandma safe," Mom said. "She'll also be with other people her age and have fun activities to keep her busy, too."

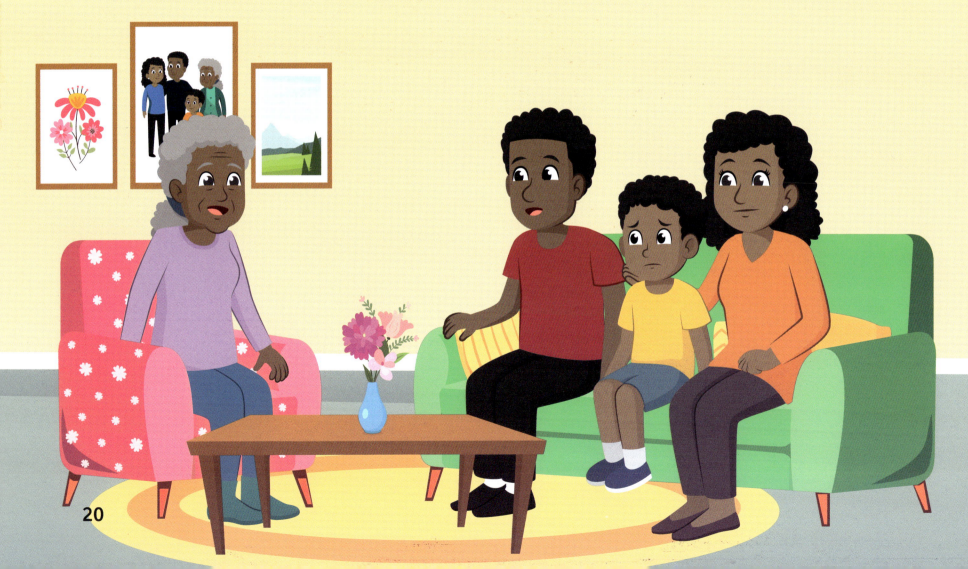

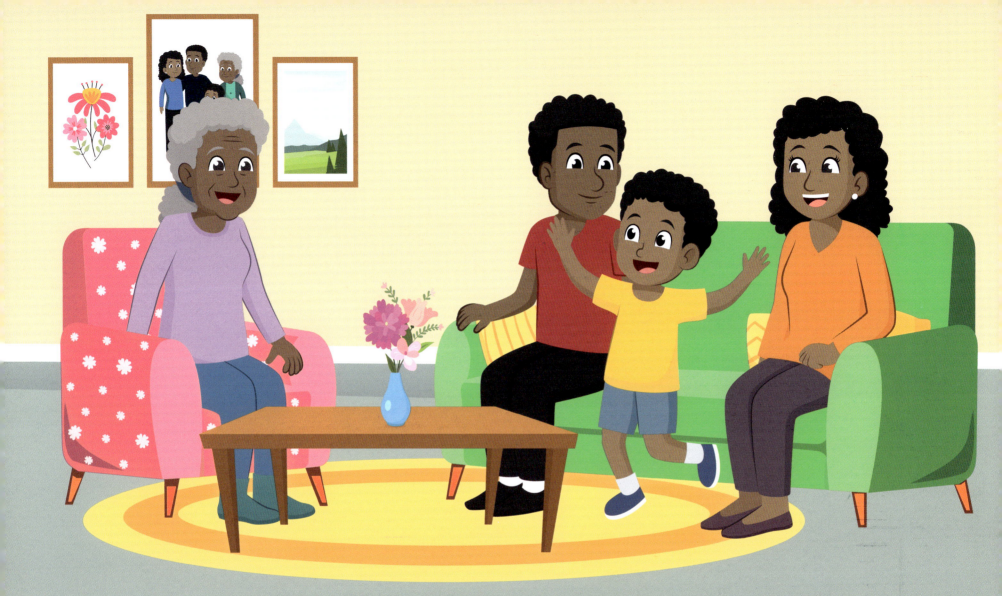

"We can visit her often," Dad assured Luke.

"We can even plant a new garden together!" Grandma added.

Luke's heart leapt at the idea that he would still be able to garden with Grandma.

A few weeks later, the family helped Grandma set up her new, lovely home. They hung pictures and moved in her favorite chair.

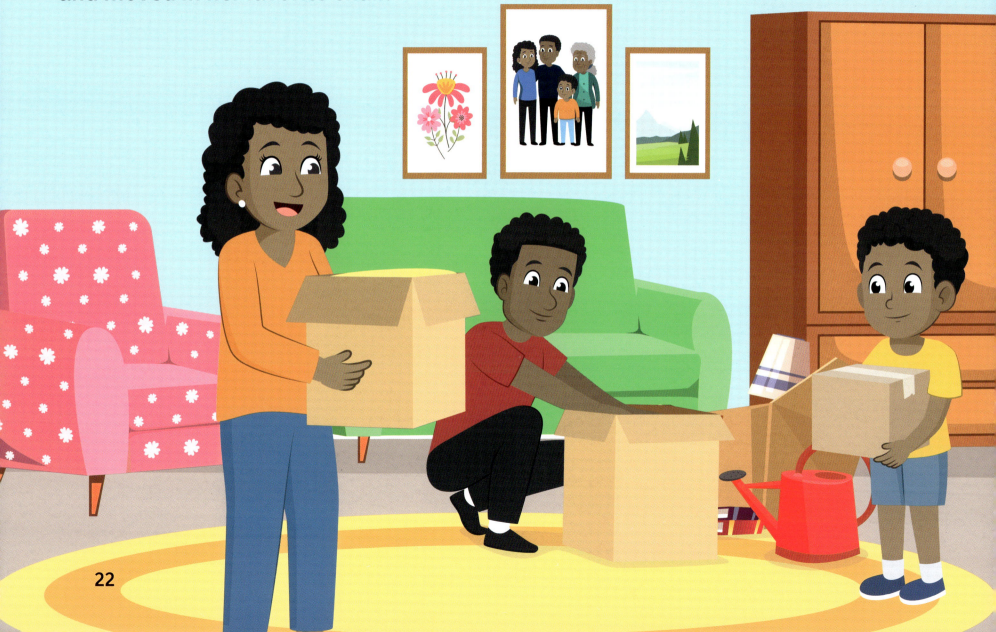

Luke even painted a picture of her favorite flowers, which brought a smile to Grandma's face.

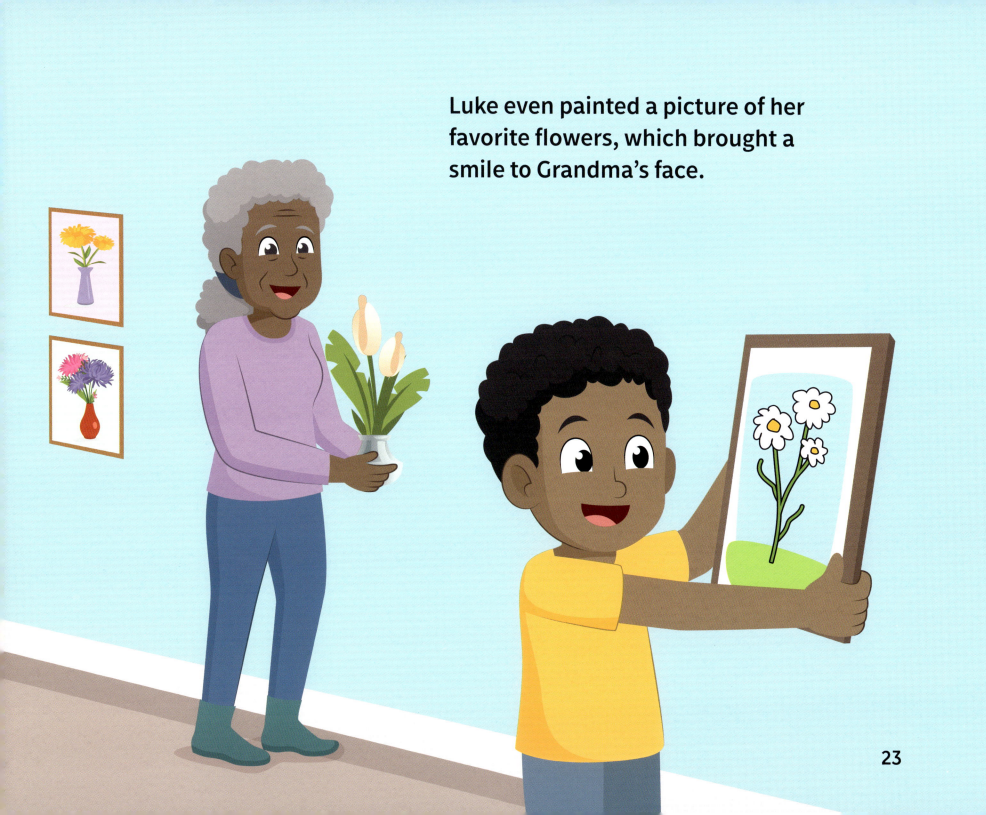

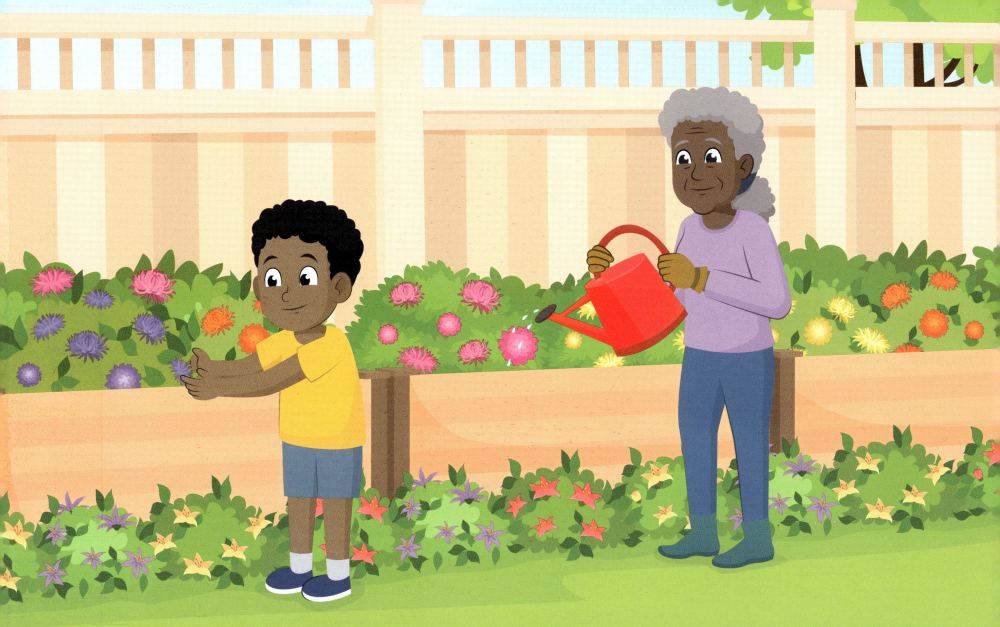

Every Sunday, Luke visited Grandma so they could garden together.

When fall arrived, they planted new flowers and cared for them.
Bursts of color replaced summer's faded blooms.

Inside, flowers decorated Grandma's windowsill. A sweet scent filled the room.

While Grandma didn't always remember Luke's name . . . or the name of her favorite flowers . . .

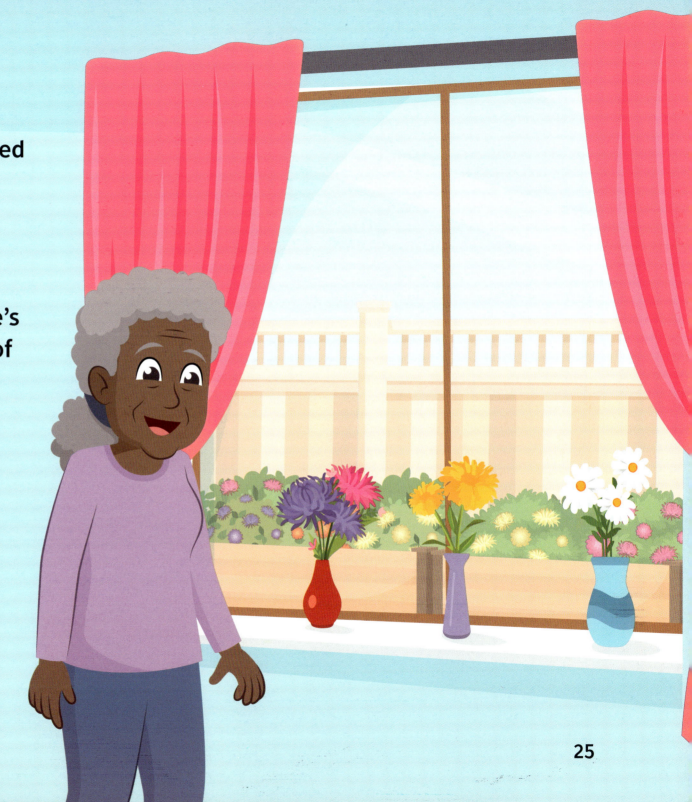

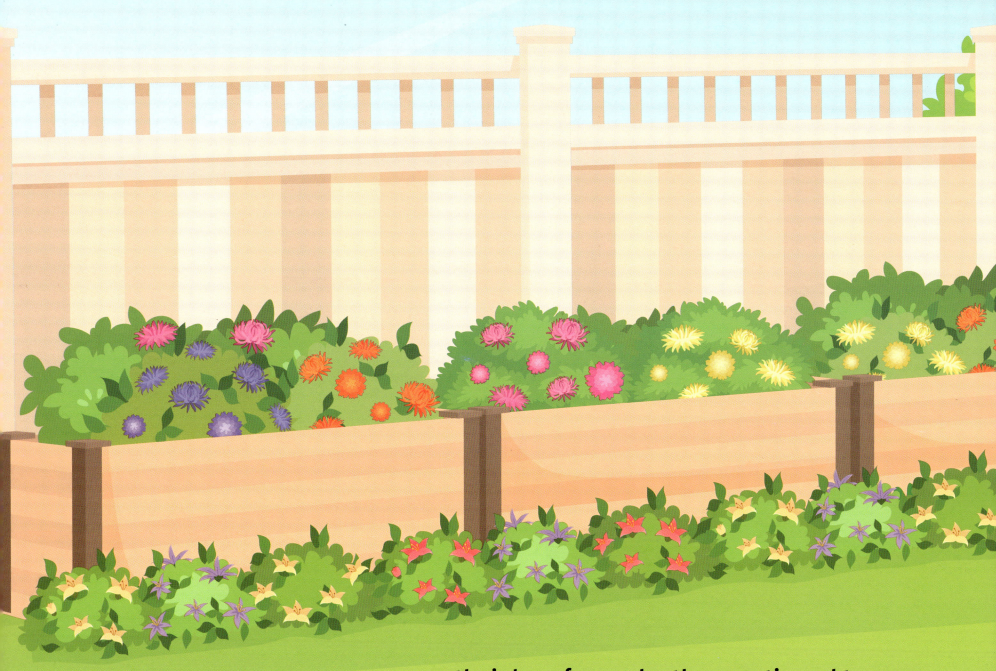

. . . their love for each other continued to grow.

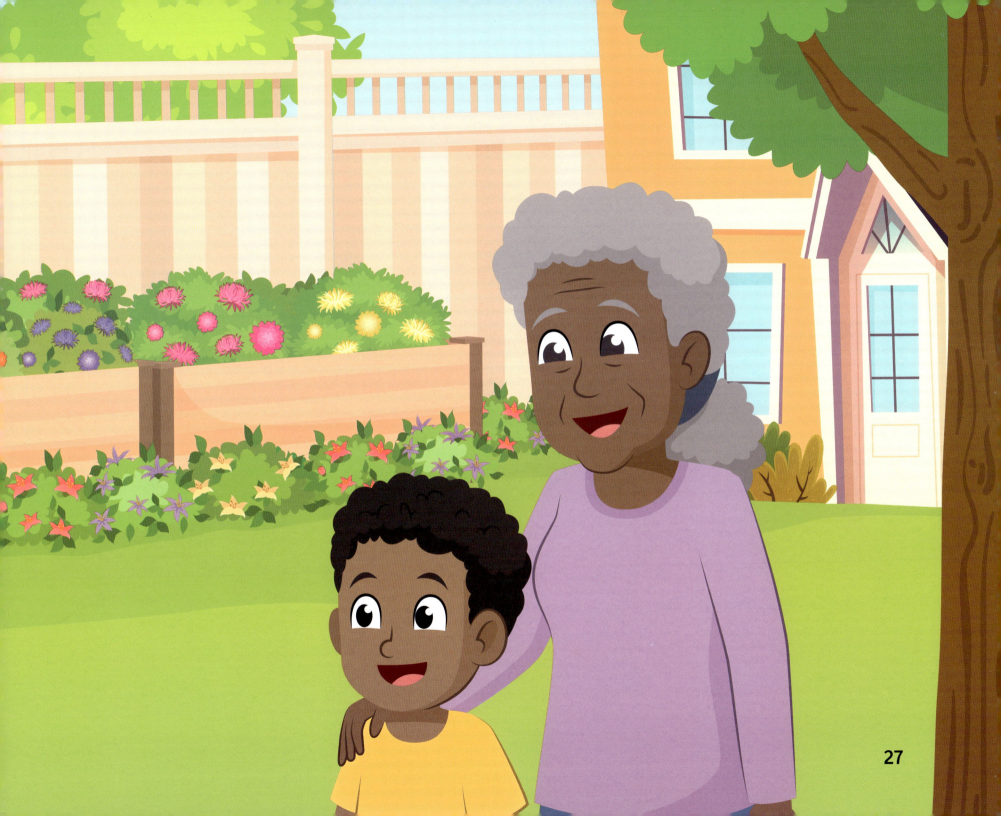

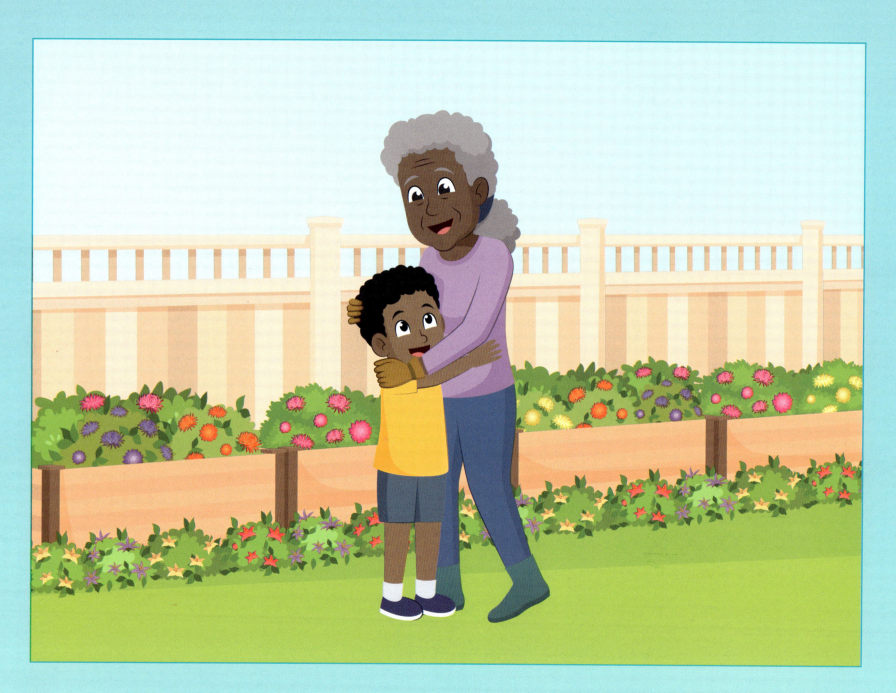

What Is Alzheimer's Disease?

Alzheimer's disease is a brain illness that affects memory, thinking, and speaking. A person may forget words, ask the same question over again, and be unable to speak clearly. They may misplace objects and not remember names or faces. They may also get frustrated and upset because of these changes.

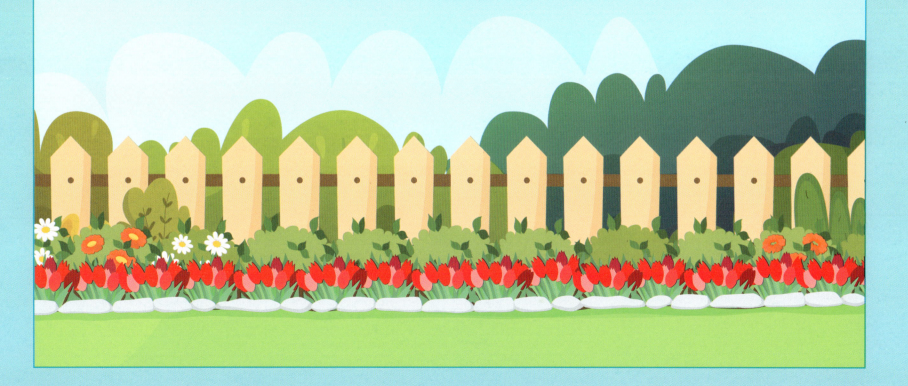

A Special Message from the Alzheimer's Foundation of America

When a family member or important friend has Alzheimer's disease, it affects everyone close to them, including children, who may have trouble understanding the changes they see, as well as dealing with their feelings about them.

AFA developed *Gardening with Grandma* as a tool to help start a conversation with a child about Alzheimer's. Often children want to hear from their person about what they are experiencing. We understand that this may not always be possible if Alzheimer's symptoms have progressed too far. A caring adult can help children formulate questions and express their concerns.

Here are some suggestions on how to begin.

Read the Book Together.

Following the story, you may want to consider some questions to invite conversation:

- *Does the grandma in the story remind you of anyone you know?*

- *Have you noticed that _____ is acting differently, too? How?*

- *How are you feeling about these changes? Listen.*

- *Do you have questions about what's going on?*

Children are highly intuitive. No doubt they have been picking up on these changes in their loved one, but they may not feel comfortable asking questions about them. It's important to welcome questioning.

Share information at a level appropriate for the age and maturity of the child. Here are some ways to describe what is going on:

- _____ *has Alzheimer's, an illness that affects memory and speaking.*

- _____ *may forget words and ask the same questions over again.*

- _____ *may not remember names or faces.*

- _____ *may also get frustrated and even upset because of these changes.*

Some Feedback to Consider.

Remind children that:

- *There are no silly questions.*

- *The person is doing the best they can and cares about them as they always did, even if they can't express it in the same way.*

- *They should not take the changes personally when their family member or friend forgets their name or repeatedly asks them the same question.*

- *The person's symptoms may change day to day and even moment to moment.*

- *It's okay to be scared.*

- *It's no one's fault.*

How to Initiate the Conversation that Includes Their Loved One

If the person with Alzheimer's is able to and feels comfortable doing so, have a conversation with them and the child together. Having the child hear from their loved one directly about what they are experiencing can be helpful.

- *Set time aside for the conversation in a comfortable setting.*

- *If possible, invite feedback from the person living with Alzheimer's about what they are experiencing.*

- *Encourage questions from your child to address with your loved one. For instance, "What can I do for you when you can't find something?" or "If you seem sad, is there anything I can do to make you feel better?"*

Be mindful that this type of conversation is more effective when the person is in the earlier stages of Alzheimer's and may not be possible in the later stages. If the person is unable to have this conversation, or feels uncomfortable doing so, do not force the issue.

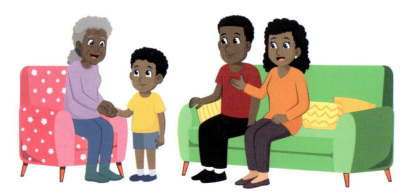

Encouraging a Child's Interaction

You may want to provide some suggestions on how to engage with their person, particularly since their loved one may be behaving differently. Some suggestions:

- *Remind the person who you are: "Hi _____, it's _____."*

- *Speak slowly. Act gently.*

- *Ask one question at a time. Wait for the person to respond.*

- *Tenderly touch their arm or hand.*

- *Let them know you've come to "share a story," "draw a picture" or "give a hug." (But always ask them first if it's okay. "Sometimes the Alzheimer's doesn't want a hug that day.")*

- *Go with the flow; each visit may be different. Let your person guide you.*

- *Try to still have fun.*

Emotional Memory

There may be a time in the Alzheimer's journey when a person with memory loss won't know the child or remember their visits. This may be difficult for the child and make them feel worried about how to engage with their loved one. Reassure the child that although their loved one may not remember a visit or a conversation, they can still hold on to the emotions they experience, carrying with them the happy and joyful feelings they felt during their time together.

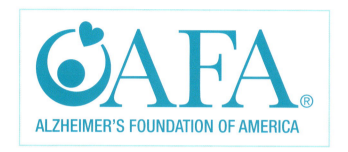

**Connect with licensed social workers and a community
who cares through the AFA Helpline, seven days a week.**

Via phone by calling 866-232-8484

Webchat by visiting www.alzfdn.org and clicking
on the chat icon in the corner of the page

Sending a text message to 646-586-5283

(The webchat and text message features are available in more than 90 languages.)